Crohn's Disease & Colitis

100 Simple Recipes for Sufferers

Brenda Webb

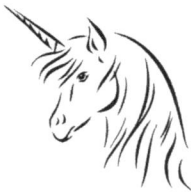

Essential Book Series

First published in Great Britain

All paper used in the printing of this book has been made from wood grown in managed, sustainable forests.

ISBN13: 978-1-78003-567-3

Essential Book Series
First published by Indepenpress Publishing Limited
25 Eastern Place
Brighton
BN2 1GJ
For Author Essentials

A catalogue record of this book is available from the British Library

Cover design © Author Essentials
info@authoressentials.com

Contents

Conversion Chart

Ounces/Grams/Milliliters

1 oz = 25g
4 oz = 100g
1lb = 450g

1 fl.oz = 30ml
5 fl.oz or 1/4pt = 150ml
20 fl.oz or 1pt =600ml

Oven Settings

130C = 250F = Gas mark 1/2
150C = 300F = Gas mark 2
180C = 350F = Gas mark 4
190C = 375F = Gas mark 5
200C = 400F = Gas mark 6
220C = 425F = Gas mark 7
230C = 450F = Gas mark 8

Spoon Measurements

1 level tablespoon flour = 15g flour
1 heaped tablespoon flour = 28g flour
1 level tablespoon sugar = 28g sugar
1 level tablespoon butter = 15g butter

Solid Measures

1 cup rice U.S = 225g rice
1 cup flour U.S = 115g flour
1 cup butter U.S = 225g butter
1 stick butter U.S = 115g butter
1 cup dried fruit U.S = 225g dried fruit
1 cup brown sugar U.S = 180g brown sugar
1 cup granulated sugar U.S = 225g granulated sugar

Liquid measures

1/4 cup	4 tablespoons	59 ml
1/3 cup	5 tablespoons + 1 teaspoon	79 ml
1/2 cup	8 tablespoons	118 ml
2/3 cup	10 tablespoons + 2 teaspoons	158 ml
3/4 cup	12 tablespoons	177 ml
7/8 cup	14 tablespoons	207 ml
1 cup	16 tablespoons	237 ml
2 cups	32 tablespoons	473 ml
4 cups	1 quart	946 ml

If you have Crohn's disease, you've come to the right place – the recipes in this cookbook were developed for healthy living with this condition.

According to Crohn's and Colitis Foundation of America, nutrition is a key principle in managing Crohn's. Foods may not cure this disease, but healthy choices can help decrease the symptoms and promote the healing of the digestive tract.

http://www.ccfa.org/resources/diet-and-nutrition-1.html

Your diet should be individualized, based on your unique nutritional needs. A nutritionist may recommend you a diet based on the parts of the bowel that are affected by this disease and the foods intolerances and allergies you may have.

However, it should be noted that all Crohn's sufferers have several nutrition related issues in common:

1) Crohn's increases your risk to become malnourished.

- Firstly, because your appetite is not so great, especially when you experience pain and during flare-ups.

- Secondly, the food is not properly assimilated, absorbed and used because Crohn's may affect various parts of the digestive tract. Research studies found multiple nutrient deficiencies associated with Crohn's – from water, proteins, fats, and carbs –to micronutrients like vitamins D, A, E, B1, B12, B6, folic acid, C, calcium, iron and zinc.

http://www.crohns.net/Miva/education/articles/Nutrient_Deficiences_in_Crohns_Disease.shtml

- Thirdly, the drugs used for the management of Chron's are also causing nutrient deficiencies. For example

– corticosteroids are necessary to decrease the inflammation of your gut; however, they deplete your body of the following nutrients: calcium, folic acid, magnesium, potassium, selenium, vitamins C, and zinc

- Lastly, the caloric (energy) needs of the body are increased in Crohn's sufferers, especially during flare-ups.

2) Crohn's is an inflammatory bowel disease.

Inflammation can involve different parts of the digestive tract's lining. This inflammation leads to abdominal pain, diarrhea and malnutrition. Luckily, there are so called "anti-inflammatory" foods that help reduce the swelling of the gut and promote the healing. Here is a sample of anti-inflammatory, Crohn's friendly diet.

Let's look at each group of foods and focus on healthy choices

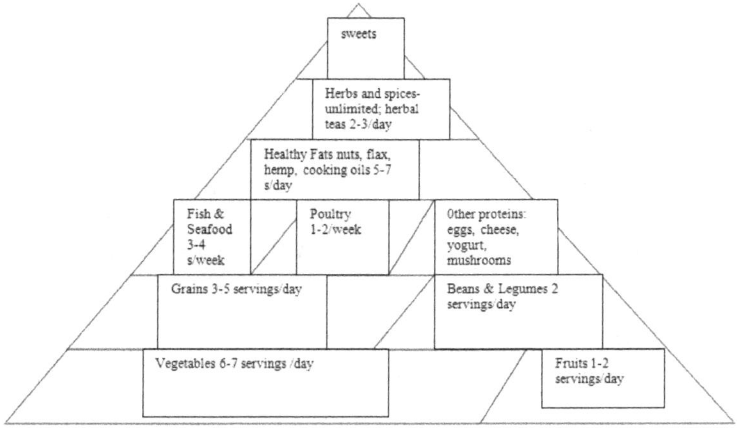
sweets
Herbs and spices-unlimited; herbal teas 2-3/day
Healthy Fats nuts, flax, hemp, cooking oils 5-7 s/day
Fish & Seafood 3-4 s/week
Poultry 1-2/week
Other proteins: eggs, cheese, yogurt, mushrooms
Grains 3-5 servings/day
Beans & Legumes 2 servings/day
Vegetables 6-7 servings /day
Fruits 1-2 servings/day

(adapted from Dr Weil's pyramid http://www.drweil.com/drw/u/ART02995/Dr-Weil-Anti-Inflammatory-Food-Pyramid.html)

Vegetables (one serving is equal to 2 cups greens, ½ cup vegetables cooked, raw or juiced) – Fresh, lightly steamed or cooked: spinach, collard greens, kale, Swiss chard, broccoli, cabbage, sauerkraut, Brussels sprouts, bell pepper, tomato, radish, kale, bok choy and cauliflower, carrots, beets, onions, scallions, leeks, peas, squashes, okra, seaweed.

Fruits (one serving = 1 fruit – like apple – or ½ cup chopped fruit or berries). Raspberries, blueberries, strawberries, Acai berries, blackberries, black mulberries, cranberries, currants, persimmons, peaches, nectarines, oranges, pink grapefruit, grapes, plums, pomegranates, blackberries, cherries, apples, pears, papaya, mango, pineapple.

Grains (one serving = ½ cup cooked grains). Brown rice, basmati rice, wild rice, buckwheat, groats, barley, quinoa, steel-cut oats, amaranth, arrowroot, buckwheat, corn, tapioca. Pasta should be cooked al dente.

Note: Many people experience great symptoms relief from removing gluten from their diets and research found that many diseases, including Crohn's are associated with gluten sensitivity. Furthermore, celiac disease (where gluten free diet is the only treatment available) shares many similarities with Crohn's and appears to be more commonly diagnosed in Crohn's sufferers compared with healthy individuals. (*** see references)

Therefore we recommend in this book many gluten free recipes. Be aware that gluten is found in wheat, barley, rye, spelt, kamut, and oats and most processed foods do contain gluten. Therefore you should cook most of your meals at home and buy only foods that are labeled "gluten free."

Beans and legumes (one serving = ½ cup cooked beans or legumes). Beans: adzuki beans, anasazi beans, black beans, black eyed beans, chickpeas, edamame (green soy beans), fava beans, lima beans, red kidney beans, lentils.

Note: Many people with Crohn's disease have troubles eating beans, because they cause excessive gas. However, beans (and meats) are an important source of proteins, and Crohn's suffers need to 30% more proteins in their diet compared with those who don't have this condition. Luckily there is a quick and easy way to cook them at home, using gas free soaking. Gas-free soak (required for all beans except lentils and black eyed peas): in a stockpot, place one pound of beans in ten cups of boiling water; boil for 2-3 minutes, cover the pot and set aside overnight. As much as 90% of the indigestible carbs that are causing gas are broken down in the soaking water. You can also add few slices of ginger to further help eliminate those gas producing sugars.

Meat, fish and other protein foods (One serving = 1 oz cheese, 1 egg, 3 oz cooked meat, 4 oz of cooked fish): cheese and yogurt, eggs, chicken, turkey, fish and seafood; replace as often as you can cow milk with goat, almond or rice milk. Mushrooms (steamed or cooked): Shiitake, enokidake, maitake, oyster, wild, and portabello mushrooms. Fermented soy (consume in small quantities): miso, tempeh, and natto.

Note: Dairy products are great sources of calcium, and this mineral is extremely important because Crohn's disease increases your risk of bone loss.

http://www.livestrong.com/article/411642-crohns-calcium/

However, most dairy products also promote inflammation and many Crohn's sufferers have intolerance to milk products. Therefore choose healthy foods like goat cheese and yogurt, and replace as much as you can cow milk with goat, almond or rice milk.

Semi-vegetarian diets are also anti-inflammatory diets – they include healthy meats such as turkey, chicken, fish and seafood and red, fatty meats are eliminated.

Remission was maintained in 94% of the cases that followed semivegetarian diet, compared with 33% in the group that followed an omnivorous diet – as indicates a small study published in 2010 in "World Journal of Gastroenterology."

http://www.livestrong.com/article/411972-healing-crohns-diet/

Healthy fats: (one serving = 1 teaspoon of oil, 2 walnuts, 1 tablespoon of flaxseed, 1 oz of nuts and seeds, flax oil, coconut oil, avocado oil, macadamia oil, olive oil – extra virgin, sesame oil)

Herbs, spices & herbal teas: Add herbs and spices, to taste: turmeric, curry powder, ginger and garlic, parsley, oregano, cilantro, basil, cinnamon, rosemary, thyme, dill, lovage(green pepper and chilli pepper – as tolerated); Herbal teas: chamomile, peppermint, licorice, ginger, white, green, oolong, jasmine teas

Sweets: dried fruits such as raisins and dates, dark or raw chocolate – as tolerated.

Don't forget to drink plenty water throughout the day.

Dealing with food intolerances and allergies

Although the list above contains healthy, anti-inflammatory foods, many people with Crohn's disease have a variety of food intolerances and allergies. These allergies are detected through elimination diets-where a person removes certain foods from diet and observes if the symptoms improve. Food allergy tests are also available.

The bottom line is that you need to track down which foods are healthy for you, and which are not. If you can't tolerate corn, you should replace corn meals with other healthy grains listed above. If you have troubles eating fibers, you should decrease the consumption of fiber rich foods.

Ideally all food you eat should be organic, if not – at least not-GMO.

This book offers you healthy, delicious recipes that contain foods with anti-inflammatory qualities and contain lots of nutrients needed by your body. We hope you'll enjoy.

• •

References

Farrell RJ, Kelly CP. Celiac sprue. *N Engl J Med.* 2002 Jan 17;346(3):180-8. Review.

http://www.huffingtonpost.com/dr-mark-hyman/gluten-what-you-dont-know_b_379089.html

http://www.ncbi.nlm.nih.gov/pubmed/15973121

http://www.ncbi.nlm.nih.gov/pubmed/20350266

http://www.ncbi.nlm.nih.gov/pubmed/22580504

http://www.ncbi.nlm.nih.gov/pubmed/20485260

http://www.ncbi.nlm.nih.gov/pubmed/19519468

Breakfast & Snack Recipes

Papaya-Banana Smoothie

Servings: 4 cups

2 cups fresh papaya chunks (optional: include few papaya seeds, crushed)

1 banana

1½ cup coconut milk

2 scoops vanilla protein powder

3-4 teaspoons freshly ground flaxseed

Preparation

In a blender, combine all of the ingredients and blend until smooth. Pour into a glass and serve. Do not add ice cubes, it is best to be consumed at room temperature.

Raspberry Mango Kale Smoothie

Servings: 4 cups

1 cup fresh raspberry

1 cup mango chunks

¼ bunch kale (leaves only)

1 banana

1½ cup almond milk

3-4 teaspoons chia seeds

Preparation

In a blender, combine all of the ingredients and blend until smooth. Pour into a glass and serve. Do not add ice cubes, it is best to be consumed at room temperature.

Carrots & Greens Smoothie

Servings: 4 cups

1 cup spinach

1 cup carrots diced

½ avocado, pitted and peeled

½ banana

1½ cup almond milk

3-4 teaspoons pumpkin seeds

Preparation

In a blender, combine all of the ingredients and blend until smooth. Pour into a glass and serve. Do not add ice cubes, it is best to be consumed at room temperature.

Quick Breakfast Raspberries

Servings: 4 cups

⅔ cup fresh raspberries
1 tablespoon honey
⅓cup cereals
¼ cup yogurt
1 tablespoon walnuts sliced
½ teaspoon ground cinnamon

Preparation

Place raspberries in a cereal bowl, add honey, cereals, yogurt and stir to combine. Sprinkle cinnamon.

Apple Cinnamon Bran Muffins

12 muffins

½ cup brown sugar
¼ cup olive oil
1 egg + 2 egg whites
¾ cup milk
2 tablespoons honey
1 cup gluten free flour
1 cups rice bran
½ cup freshly ground flax seeds
1½ teaspoons baking powder
dash of salt
½ teaspoon ground cinnamon
1 chopped apples

Preparation

1. Preheat oven to 400°F (204°C).

2. Mix brown sugar and olive oil in a medium bowl; Add egg and white eggs and beat until well blended. Add milk and honey

3. Mix flour, rice bran, flax seeds, baking powder, salt, and cinnamon in a bowl. Add milk mixture to flour mixture. Stir in apples.

4. Spoon batter evenly into prepared muffin cups. Bake at 400°F for 15-20 minutes.

Rhubarb Tart

6 servings

2 cups gluten free mix flour
a dash of salt
1 cup brown sugar
2 tablespoons honey
14 tablespoons of coconut oil, melted
1 pound fresh rhubarb, diced
1 cups fresh blueberries
cooking spray

Preparation

Heat oven to 400°F (204°C)

1. Mix the flour, salt, and 2 tablespoons of the honey in a food processor

2. Add the coconut oil and water and mix until the dough comes together

3. Place the dough and roll it onto a lightly floured surface.

4. Place the dough in an oven pan coated with cooking spray. Let the dough to hang slightly over the edge. Top with the rhubarb and sugar. Fold the dough's over rhubarb and blueberries.

5. Bake at 400°F. until golden brown (50 to 55 minutes).

Breakfast Chicken Tortillas

4 servings

4 medium rice tortillas
8 oz (225 grams) breast chicken cooked and sliced
3 eggs
cooking spray
¼ cup goat cheese
¼ cup medium Salsa
¼ cup yogurt
1 tablespoon parsley leaves, finely chopped
salt and pepper, to taste

Preparation

Heat oven to 250°F (121°C)

1. Place tortillas in an oven tray, in the oven for 10 minutes.

2. Put the olive oil in a saucepan over medium heat.

3. Add the eggs and chicken breast and stir with a spatula to scramble until the eggs are cooked

4. Spread the goat cheese on tortillas. Add the chicken-egg mixture, parsley and add salt and pepper to taste. Roll up the tortillas. Serve with salsa and yogurt.

Egg, Avocado, and Tuna Pitas

4 servings

1 cup tuna, canned
½ cup mild salsa
¼ cup goat cheese
salt and pepper, to taste
2 pitas (see the gluten free pita recipe)
2 hard-cooked large eggs, sliced
½ avocado, sliced
1 cup baby spinach

Preparation

Heat oven to 250°F (121°C)

1. Place tortillas in an oven tray, in the oven – for 10 minutes.

2. Open pita halves and coat each half with goat cheese and baby spinach

3. Add tuna, eggs, salsa, avocado. Add salt and pepper to taste

Gluten (and Yeast) Free Pita

2 pitas

1 egg
¼ cup of water
1 tablespoon oil
⅓ cup almond or rice flour
⅛ teaspoon baking soda
⅛ teaspoon salt
1 tablespoon flax seeds
cooking spray

Preparation

1. Preheat oven to 350°F.

2. Combine egg, water and oil, using a whisk.

3. Add flour, backing soda, salt and flax seeds

4. Use ½ of the mixture-pour onto an oven tray coated with cooking spray in a round shape; add the second ½ of the mixture the same way

5. Bake this mixture at 350°F until slightly crisp (15-20 minutes)

6. Let cool, cut in half and slice down the center with a knife to create the pocket

Falafel with Beans, Cheese and Avocado

4 servings

1 can mixed beans, rinsed and drained
4 tablespoons goat cheese
2 tablespoons green onions, chopped
1 clove garlic, crushed
1 teaspoon coriander
⅛ teaspoon ground cumin
1 large egg
1 teaspoons olive oil

Spread:

¼ cup mashed avocado

2 tablespoons tomato paste

2 tablespoons yogurt

1 teaspoon lime juice

salt and pepper, to taste

Other ingredients:

2 pitas

mixed green salad

Preparation

Mix the beans in a food processor. Place the bean mixture into a bowl. Add goat cheese, green onions, garlic, coriander, cumin and egg and mix them well with a wooden spoon. Divide this mixture into 4 small balls.

Add the balls to a heated sauce pan, coated with cooking spray and cook until golden brown (around 5 minutes).

Spread: mix avocado, tomato paste, yogurt, lime juice and salt.

Spread avocado mixture into each half pita. Place 1 small ball in each pita half and add the mixed greens salad.

Egg Burritos

2 burritos

2 eggs and 2 white eggs
1 tablespoon water
1 teaspoon fresh parsley, chopped
salt and pepper, to taste
½ teaspoon olive oil
4 tablespoons goat cheese
2 medium tortillas
¼ cup red bell peppers, chopped
2 tablespoons medium salsa

Preparation

1. Mix the eggs, white eggs, water, parsley, salt and pepper in a bowl, with a whisk.

2. Add the mixture to a pan coated with cooking oil, and bring to a heat. Stir with a wooden spoon to scramble, until the eggs are cooked.

3. Spread the 2 tablespoons goat cheese down the center of each tortilla; add ½ of the egg mixture, ½ of bell peppers, parsley and salsa. Roll up the burrito and repeat this step to make the second burrito.

Roasted Pepper-Chickpea Hummus

3 garlic cloves

juice from 2 limes

⅓ cup tahini

1 tablespoon olive oil

salt and pepper, to taste

2 cups chickpeas, canned, drained

1 cup of roasted peppers

4 pitas, cut in quarters

fresh parsley leaves, chopped

Preparation

Heat 1 tablespoon oil in a small pan over medium heat. Add garlic; cook 30 seconds.

In a food processor, combine chickpeas, tahini and lime juice. Process until smooth. Add red peppers and roasted garlic and contiue to mix. Serve with pita. Sprinkle with fresh parsley.

Cumin-Mixed Beans Hummus

1 tablespoon olive oil

3 garlic cloves

1 tablespoon curry powder

½ teaspoon cumin seeds

½ cup yogurt

salt and pepper, to taste

2 cups canned mixed beans, canned, drained

4 pitas, cut in quarters

Preparation

1. Heat 1 tablespoon oil in a small pan over medium heat. Add garlic and cook 30 seconds.

2. In a food processor, combine garlic mixture with mixed beans, yogurt, curry and cumin. Process until smooth. Serve with pita.

Sundried Tomato & Chickpea Hummus

¼ cup cashews, finely chopped

½ cup chickpeas canned

⅓ cup Tomatoes, sundried, chopped

lime juice from 2 limes

pinch of salt

½ cup water

1 tablespoon fresh parsley leaves

2 tablespoons olive oil

one bag of rice crackers

Preparation

In a blender, add the water first, then olive oil, chickpeas, sundried tomatos, cashews, lime juice, ½ tablespoon parsley and salt. Blend well until this mixture becomes creamy.

Sprinkle with the remaining parsley leaves and serve with rice crackers

Gluten Free Pancakes

6 pancakes

¾ cups almond milk
½ cup pumpkin puree, unsweetened
2 eggs
1 tablespoon coconut oil
½ teaspoon vanilla extract
1 cup gluten-free all purpose flour
1½ tablespoons brown sugar
pinch of salt
1 teaspoon baking powder (gluten free)
½ teaspoon baking soda
1 teaspoon cinnamon
⅛ teaspoon guar gum
1 tablespoon flax seeds
cooking oil
Topping: 6 tablespoons maple syrup

Preparation

Mix together almond milk, pumpkin puree, eggs, oil and vanilla in a bowl, using a whisk, until the mixture is creamy.

In a second bowl mix flour, sugar, baking powder, baking soda, salt, flax seeds and guar gum with a whisk. Add the pumpkin mixture and stir well.

Heat a cooking pan coated with cooking spray. Pour ¼ cup of batter into the pan, and cook 2-3 minutes on each side. Serve with maple syrup.

Potato Pancakes

6 pancakes

4 large potatoes, peeled and shredded

4 eggs

1 cup cheddar cheese, shredded

½ tablespoon onion finely chopped

1 garlic clove, finely chopped

salt and pepper, to taste

cooking oil

2 tablespoon fresh parsley, chopped

6 tablespoons yogurt

Preparation

In a bowl, mix potatoes with eggs, cheese, onion, garlic, salt and pepper.

Heat a cooking pan coated with cooking spray. Pour ¼ cup of the mixture into the pan, and cook few minutes(until browned) on each side. Serve each pancake with one tablespoon of yogurt and sprinkle with parsley

Lunch and Dinner

Soups

Chicken Pasta Soup

10 servings (serving size: 1 cup)

2¼ cups (6 oz) gluten free pasta

Cooking spray

¾ pound breast chicken chunks

1 cup chopped onion

3 cups tomato sauce

parsley leaves

2 cups chicken broth (see the recipe for home made broth)

1 cups canned kidney beans

Preparation

1. Cook pasta according to package directions. Do not add salt or butter/oil. Drain.

2. Place the cooking pot over medium-high heat until hot. Coat it with cooking spray. Add chicken and onion; cook over medium heat until meat is browned.

3. Add cooked pasta, tomato sauce, beans and broth. Cook 10 minutes or until thoroughly heated.

Baked Potato Soup

10 servings (cups)

4 baking potatoes
⅔ cup gluten free flour
6 cups low-fat milk
1 cup shredded mozzarella cheese
1 teaspoon salt
1 cup low fat sour cream
¾ cup chopped green onions
2 tablespoons chopped fresh parsley
½ teaspoon dried thyme

Preparation

1. Preheat oven to 400°F (204°C). Bake potatoes until tender. Cool, peel and mash them.

2. Place flour in a pot; add milk, stirring with a whisk until blended. Cook until the mixture becomes thick. Add mashed potatoes, ¾ cup of mozzarella cheese and salt and stir until cheese melts.

3. Stir in sour cream, ½ cup onions and dried thyme. Cook until thoroughly heated. Sprinkle each serving with cheese, onion, and fresh parsley.

Turkey-Egg Noodle Soup

4 servings (8 cups)

Cooking spray

1 cup shredded carrots

¾ cup chopped onion

1 cup shredded celery root

¼ teaspoon salt

6 cups chicken broth

2 cups uncooked egg noodles

2 cups shredded cooked turkey

2 tablespoons chopped fresh parsley

Preparation

Heat a large saucepan over medium-high heat, coat it with cooking spray. Add carrot, onion and sauté until onion is lightly browned; add carrots and celery and sauté few more minutes. Add broth and noodles; bring to a boil. Add shredded turkey and cook few more minutes minutes. Sprinkle with fresh parsley leaves.

Tomato Soup

8 servings (8 cups)

2 tablespoons oil
1 cup chopped onion
2 cups fresh or frozen vegetables: diced carrots, corn and peas
1½ cups vegetable broth
1 teaspoon fresh basil
1 can diced canned tomatoes
¾ cup tomato sauce
1 cup 2% fat yogurt

Preparation

1. Place the olive oil in a soup pot over medium-high heat. Add onion, carrots, corn and peas; sauté until tender. Add broth, ½ teaspoon basil, tomatoes sauce and tomatoes; bring to a boil. Reduce heat; simmer 15 minutes.

2. Place ½ of the mixture in a blender, and process until smooth. Repeat procedure with remaining ½ of the mixture. Add the yogurt and sprinkle with basil.

Minestrone Soup

6 servings

1¼ cups canned black eyed beans

3 tablespoons olive oil

2 medium shallots, minced

4 cloves garlic, minced

2 large celery sticks, diced

2 medium carrots, diced

2 tablespoons tomato paste

1 cup diced tomatoes – canned

1 cup chicken broth

Salt and pepper, to taste

½ cup fresh parsley leaves

lime juice

Preparation

In a soup pot, heat 2 tablespoons of the oil. Add the shallots, celery and carrot and cook until softened. Add the garlic and cook for a few more minutes. Add the tomato paste, tomatoes and broth; bring to a boil. Remove the pan from the stove, and let this mixture cool for 45 min – 1 hour. Add the beans, salt and enough water to thin out the soup. Sprinkle with fresh parsley leaves; add lime if desired.

Red Kidney Bean Soup

4 servings

3 tablespoon olive oil

3 6-inch corn tortillas, cut into narrow wedges

2 cups of red kidney beans – canned

1 medium onion, diced

1 teaspoon ground cumin

1 tablespoon of chopped lovage

salt and pepper to taste

rice crackers

Preparation

In a soup pot, heat olive oil. Add the onion and cook until softened. Add the cumin, the beans and 2 cups of water. Bring to a simmer and cook until thickened. Add lovage and salt. Serve with rice crackers.

Seafood Soup

6 servings

2 tablespoons olive oil
1 medium onion, finely chopped
¼ cup shredded celery root
1 medium carrot, shredded
2 cloves garlic, chopped
2 teaspoons coriander seeds

1 cup whole tomatoes, chopped and juices reserved
1 lb frozen seafood mix
Salt and pepper to taste
lime juice

Preparation

In a soup pot, heat the oil. Add the onion and cook until softened. Add the garlic, shredded carrots and celery and coriander seeds and cook until fragrant. Stir in the tomato paste, the tomatoes and bring to a boil. Add the frozen seafood mix, cover partially and simmer for 45 minutes. Add some lime juice if desired.

Avocado Chicken Soup

⅓ cup quinoa

1⅓ cups water

Salt and pepper, to taste

1 pound (½ kg) skinless chicken breast

1 medium onion, sliced

2 cloves garlic, chopped

2 medium carrots, finely diced

1 cup of frozen corn

½ cup chopped cilantro

8 cups chicken broth

½ pound potatoes, peeled and diced

1 avocado, peeled, pitted & diced

½ cup low fat yogurt

Preparation

1. Place quinoa (⅓ cup) in a small saucepan with water (⅔ cup). Bring to a boil, cover, and simmer over low heat. Simmer until all liquid is absorbed. Remove from heat and let stand for 5 minutes.

2. In a soup pot, mix the chicken, onion, garlic, corn, carrots, potatoes and the cilantro with the chicken broth. Add salt and pepper and bring to a boil. Simmer the mixture until the chicken is cooked through. Add the quinoa.

3. Ladle the soup into bowls and add the avocado, yogurt; sprinkle with cilantro.

Lentil Soup

6 servings

1 tablespoon olive oil

1 small onion

1 cup tomatoes, diced

2 potatoes, peeled and diced

1 bunch kale leaves

½ cup brown lentils

salt and pepper

¼ fresh parsley leaves

¼ cup low fat yogurt

Preparation

In a soup pot, heat the oil. Add the onion and cook until softened; add tomatoes and cook for two minutes. Add 6 cups of water and bring to a boil. Add the potatoes, kale, lentils, salt and pepper. Simmer until the lentils are tender. Remove the pan from heat.

Ladle the soup into bowls; add the yogurt and sprinkle with parsley.

Pumpkin Soup

8 servings

2 tablespoons olive oil

1 large onion, chopped

3 garlic cloves, minced

1 cup pumpkin puree

4 cups chicken broth

1 cup croutons

¼ tablespoon cinnamon

a dash of nutmeg

1 cup of low fat milk

Salt and pepper

Preparation

In a soup pot, heat the oil over medium heat. Add the onion and garlic and cook until softened. Add the pumpkin puree and broth. Bring to a boil, stirring occasionally. Stir in milk, nutmeg, cinnamon, salt and pepper, simmer for 5 minutes. Remove from heat and puree in a blender. Ladle the soup into bowls and serve with croutons.

Pea Soup with Dill

6 servings (cups)

3 tablespoons olive oil
1 medium onion, chopped
2 cups vegetable broth
3 cups peas (fresh or frozen)
½ cup low fat yogurt
salt and pepper
2 tablespoons dill

Preparation

In a soup pot, heat 2 tablespoons olive oil over medium heat. Add onion and cook until softened. Add broth, 2 cups of water and bring to a boil. Add peas and simmer until cooked.

Working in batches, transfer the mixture to a blender; add one tablespoon dill, one tablespoon olive oil, yogurt, salt and pepper.

Ladle the soup into bowls and sprinkle with dill.

Squash Soup with Tortilla Chips

8 servings

2 tablespoon olive oil
1 medium squash (peeled, seeded, and diced)
1 cup carrots diced
1 cup sweet potatoes , diced
1 small onion, chopped
¼ cup yogurt
salt and pepper

Preparation

In a soup pot, heat olive oil over medium heat. Add onion and cook until softened. Add squash, carrot, and potatoes and sauté (10-15 minutes). Add 3 cups of water and bring to a boil. Transfer the mixture to a food processor; add yogurt, salt and pepper.

Ladle the soup into bowls. Serve with tortilla chips.

Thai Chicken Soup

10 servings (cups)

4 cups water
3 cups kale leaves (fresh or frozen)
1 cup peas (fresh or frozen)
1 small pack thai noodles
1 tablespoon olive oil
¼ cup shallots, sliced
2 teaspoons curry powder
½ teaspoon ground coriander
2 garlic cloves, chopped
6 cups water
1 pound shredded cooked chicken breast
½ cup green onions, chopped
salt and pepper
two limes

Preparation

1. Bring 4 cups water to a boil in a pot. Add noodles and cook for few minutes. Drain.

2. Heat olive oil in a soup pot over medium heat. Add shallots, kale and peas; sauté 1 minute, stirring constantly. Add 7 cups of water to pan, and bring to a boil. Add chicken, green onions, curry, coriander, salt, pepper and cook few more minutes. Pour chicken mixture over noodle mixture in bowls. Serve with lime wedges.

Garden Vegetable Soup

8 servings

2 tablespoons olive oil

2 garlic cloves, minced

2 cups carrots, diced

2 cups potatoes, diced

2 cups green beans

2 cups tomatoes, diced

1 cup corn kernels

1 small onion, chopped

salt and pepper, to taste

½ teaspoon freshly ground black pepper

2 tablespoons chopped fresh parsley leaves

1 to 2 teaspoons lime juice

Preparation

In a soup pot, heat olive oil over medium-high heat. Add onions and garlic, cook until soften. Add salt and 8 cups of water and bring to a boil. Add the carrots, potatoes, tomatoes, corn kernels, and green beans and continue to cook until soften.

Ladle the soup into bowls, sprinkle with parsley. Add lemon juice and black pepper if desired.

Tortellini Soup

6 servings

1 lb (½ kg) breast chicken, cut into small strips
6 cups water
2 carrots, diced
½ medium celery root, sliced
one small onion, chopped
½ bunch kale leaves
1 9-oz pack gluten free tortellini
salt and pepper
salt and pepper
2 tablespoons fresh parsley, chopped

Preparation

In a soup pan add 3 cups of water. Bring to a boil. Add tortellini and cook according to the package directions. Drain.

In a large stock pot, heat olive oil over medium-high heat. Add the onion and cook until soften. Add 8 cups of water. Bring to a boil. Add the chicken strips, carrots, celery root, and kale leaves. Add tortellini when chicken is cooked, salt and pepper.

Ladle the soup into bowls and sprinkle with the parsley leaves.

Broccoli Soup

Serves 4

1 tablespoon olive oil
½ onion, chopped
1 bunch broccoli sliced
1large potato, peeled and diced
½ cup of carrots, diced
 salt and pepper
rice crackers
½ cup yogurt
1 tablespoon parsley leaves, chopped

Preparation

In a soup pot, heat olive oil over medium-high heat. Add the onion and cook until soften. Add 4 cups of water, broccoli, potatoes, carrots, salt and pepper. Cook until vegetables are tender.

Transfer the mixture to a blender; add yogurt, salt and pepper. Ladle the soup into bowls and sprinkle with parsley leaves. Serve with rice crackers.

Chickpea Soup

Serves 4

1 4-lb chicken, skinless, boneless, cut into small strips

1 cup carrots, diced

4 celery stalks, diced

1 medium onion, chopped

salt and pepper

⅓ cup quinoa

1 cup kalamata olives, pitted and chopped

1 cup of canned chickpeas, drained and rinsed

2 tablespoons of parsley, chopped

Preparation

Place quinoa in a small saucepan with water (⅔ cup water for ⅓ cup quinoa). Bring to a boil, cover, and simmer over low heat. Simmer until all liquid is absorbed. Remove from heat and let stand for 5 minutes. Add the olives.

In a large soup pot, heat olive oil over medium-high heat. Add the onion and cook until softened. Add 4 cups of water and bring to a boil. Add chicken strips, carrots, celery, salt and pepper. Cook until vegetables are tender. Add chickpeas and simmer few more minutes.

Ladle the soup over the quinoa and olive mixture. Sprinkle with parsley.

Carrot Soup

4 servings

1 tablespoon olive oil

1 medium onion, sliced

2 cups carrots, diced

½ cup celery root, grated

1 cup of red bell peppers, sliced

1 tablespoon ginger, grated

salt and pepper

½ cup low fat yogurt

2 tablespoons fresh dill, chopped

Preparation

In a large soup pot, heat olive oil over medium-high heat. Add the onion and cook until softened. Add 4 cups of water and bring to a boil. Stir in the carrots, bell peppers, celery and ginger. Simmer until the carrots are tender.

Transfer the mixture to a blender; add yogurt, salt and pepper. Ladle the soup into bowls and sprinkle with fresh dill.

Mushroom Millet Soup

4 servings

½ cup millet
1½ tablespoons olive oil
1 medium onions, sliced
1 cup of carrots, diced
1 cup of celery stalks, diced
2 cups of *Portobello mushroom,* sliced
2 teaspoons of thyme leaves, chopped
salt and pepper
optional: ½ cup low fat yogurt

Preparation

In a saucepan, bring 2 cups of water to a boil. Add millet and ½ tablespoon olive oil. Stir frequently. Cover and simmer over medium heat until millet becomes fluffy and the water is absorbed.

In a soup pot, heat 1 tablespoon olive oil over medium-low heat. Add the onion and cook until softened. Add the carrots, celery and the mushrooms, and cook, covered, until all vegetables are tender. Add 5 cups of water, thyme, salt and pepper and simmer.

Ladle the soup over the millet. Add low fat yogurt if desired.

Home Made Vegetable Broth

6 cups of mixed vegetables: mushrooms, onions, leeks, carrots, celery, broccoli, zucchini, bell peppers, tomatoes

2 bay leaves

2 garlic cloves, sliced

½ tablespoon of rosemary

½ tablespoon of thyme

Preparation

Add all ingredients to large stockpot. Cover the vegetables with water and bring to a boil over high heat. Reduce temperature and simmer for 1-2 hours.

Let this vegetable mixture cool, then strain and discard the vegetables (which can be used for lunch or dinner) Pour broth into jars. Store up to five days in fridge.

Home Made Chicken Broth

4 cups of mixed vegetables: onions, leeks, carrots, celery stalks

2 pounds of skinless bony chicken

2 bay leaves

2 garlic cloves, sliced

1 tablespoon of Italian mixed herbs (basil, rosemary, oregano)

Preparation

Add all ingredients to large stockpot. Cover the vegetables with water and bring to a boil over high heat. Reduce temperature and simmer for 1-2 hours.

Let this vegetable mixture cool, then strain and discard the chicken and vegetables (which can be used for lunch or dinner) Pour broth into jars. Store up to five days in fridge.

Chicken & Peppers Stew

6 servings (6 cups)

2 teaspoons olive oil
1 cup onion, chopped
1 pound skinless, boneless chicken thighs, cut into strips
2 cups of mixed bell peppers (green, red and yellow)
2 cups potatoes, diced
½ cup eggplants, diced
1½ cups carrots, diced
1 teaspoon dried oregano
salt and pepper
2 garlic cloves, minced
2 cups home made chicken broth (or water)
4 teaspoons chopped fresh cilantro

Preparation

In a stock pot, heat 1 tablespoon olive oil over medium-low heat. Add the onion and chicken and cook until softened. Add potatoes, carrots, eggplants, broth (or water) and bring to a boil. Cover, reduce temperature and simmer until vegetables are tender. Add bell peppers, and oregano, stirring occasionally until softened.

Ladle the stew into bowls and sprinkle with cilantro.

Avocado Soup with Pumpkin Seeds

4 servings

2 ripe avocados, peeled, pitted & diced

2 cups low fat yogurt

1⅓ cups vegetable broth

½ cup carrots, finely diced

½ cup leeks

1 clove garlic, minced

1 green bell pepper, sliced

4 tablespoons pumpkin seeds

2 teaspoons olive oil

lemon wedges

salt and pepper to taste

cooking spray

Preparation

In a stock pot, heat 1 tablespoon olive oil over medium-low heat. Add the leeks, carrots and green pepper and cook until softened. Add vegetable broth and bring to a boil.

Remove the pot from heat, and let it cool for 15 minutes. Place this mixture in a blender and add yogurt and fresh avocados, until it is well blended and smooth.

Add salt and pepper, one tablespoon of oil and sprinkle with pumpkin seeds and lemon wedges.

Salads and Appetizers

Spinach Salad

4 servings

3 cups baby spinach leaves

1 cup Portobello mushrooms

2 tablespoons fresh parsley, chopped

salt and pepper to taste

2 tablespoons fresh lime juice

2 tablespoons olive oil

2 tablespoons chia seeds

Preparation

In a small cup mix the lime juice with olive oil, chia seeds and parsley.

Place the spinach leaves on each salad plates. Top each with ¼ cup mushrooms, then add the oil-lime-chia-parsley mixture. Add salt and pepper to taste.

Tomato Salad

4 servings

5 tomatoes, diced

1 green onion, chopped

½ cup chopped fresh basil

1 garlic clove, chopped

salt and pepper, to taste

2 tablespoons balsamic vinegar + 2 tablespoons olive oil OR ½ cup yogurt

Preparation

Mix tomatoes and cucumber in a bowl. Add the garlic, cucumbers and green onion. Add salt and pepper to taste. Drizzle with balsamic vinegar and olive oil or replace this dressing with yogurt. Place the mixture on each salad plates. Sprinkle with fresh basil.

Sauerkraut Salad

6 servings

2 tablespoons balsamic vinegar

2 tablespoons olive oil

2 cups of sauerkraut, drained

½ cup carrots, shredded

½ cup celery root, shredded

2 tablespoons freshly ground flax seeds

Preparation

Mix sauerkraut, carrots and celery root in a bowl. Add the vinegar, then the oil and blend thoroughly. Chill few hours before serving. Sprinkle with flax seeds.

Okra Salad

4-6 servings

4 cups fresh okra
1 green onion, chopped
1 red bell pepper, diced
1 tomato, diced
2 tablespoons of balsamic vinegar
2 tablespoons olive oil
2 tablespoons pine nuts

Preparation

Place the okra in a pan over medium heat. Cook until tender (around 5 minutes) Transfer the okra to a bowl, and mix with the onion, pepper, and tomato. Pour vinegar and oil over the salad and toss to combine. Top with pine nuts and serve.

Fresh Cabbage Salad with Avocado Dressing

4 servings

2 cups green cabbage, finely shredded
½ cup carrots, shredded

Dressing:
¾ cups of dressing
¼ cup orange juice
¼ cup lime juice
1 tablespoon yogurt
1 large avocado, peeled and diced
salt and pepper to taste

Preparation

Place the lime juice, orange juice, salt, yogurt and avocado in blender and blend until smooth. Refrigerate until ready to serve.

Salad

Mix the green cabbage and carrots in a bowl. Top with avocado dressing and serve.

Kale Salad

4 servings

1 fresh kale bunch, ribs removed, shredded
2 tablespoons balsamic vinegar
2 tablespoons lime juice
Salt and pepper, to taste
1 orange, peeled and diced
4 tablespoons cottage cheese

Preparation

Mix the kale with orange in a bowl. Add vinegar, lime juice, salt and pepper and toss to combine. Top with cottage cheese and serve.

Summer Salad

Serve 4

2 cups of mixed green salad

2 tomatoes, diced

1 avocado, diced

1 orange bell pepper, sliced

½ cup of pecans, chopped

¼ cup cranberries, dried, unsweetened

2 tablespoons fresh lime juice

2 tablespoons avocado oil

2 tablespoons of sesame seeds

salt and pepper to taste

Preparation

In a bowl add the mixed greens. Add with tomatoes, avocado and bell pepper and combine. Add the lime juice first, then avocado oil, salt and pepper and stir to combine. Top with pecans and cranberries.

Heat a small pan (dry, without cooking oil) over medium heat. Pour the sesame seeds, so they form a thin layer and cook them for 2-3 minutes (until they become golden brown), while stirring with an wooden spoon. Remove from heat and sprinkle them on the salad.

Potato Salad

3 eggs

2 pounds potatoes peeled and diced

salt and pepper

3 tablespoons balsamic vinegar

1 tablespoon olive oil

½ small red onion, chopped

½ cup pickles

1 cup of red peppers

½ cup flat-leaf parsley leaves

½ teaspoon mild mustard

Preparation

1. Put eggs in a pot and cover with cold water. Bring to a boil. *Cut* the *cooled hard boiled eggs* into *slices*.

2. Place potatoes in a large pot, cover with water, and bring to a boil. Reduce the temperature and cook until tender. Drain potatoes, add salt.

3. Finely chop onion, celery, red bell peppers, pickles, and parsley in a bowl. Add this mixture to potatoes, then add the eggs, mustard, balsamic vinegar and olive oil. Sprinkle with fresh parsley .

*you can also steam the peppers, onion and celery.

Grilled Pepper-Zucchini Salad

6 servings

4 medium peppers (one yellow, one orange, one red and one green) halved and seeded

1 zucchini sliced

½ eggplant sliced

¼ cup tomatoes, sun-dried and chopped

1 tablespoon olive oil

1 tablespoon vinegar balsamic

salt and pepper, to taste

one teaspoon parsley leaves, dried

Preparation

1. Grill peppers, zucchini and eggplant on medium-high until soft.

2. When cool enough to handle, chop the vegetables into cubes and place them in a bowl. Add sun-dried tomatoes, oil, vinegar and salt. Sprinkle with parsley.

Appetizers & Main Dishes

Cheese & Olives Appetizer

6 servings

½ French bread loaf

2 tablespoons yogurt

1garlic clove, crushed

1 cup cedar cheese, shredded

½ cup green olives, sliced

½ cup tomatoes, diced

1 tablespoon fresh parsley leaves

Preparation

Heat the oven at 300ºF. Cut the bread into small slices and place them in an oven pan coated with cooking spray.

In a bowl, mix the garlic, cheese, green olive and tomatoes.

Spread this mixture onto bread slices. Bake until cheese is melted (around 3-5 minutes).

Remove the pan from oven, add yogurt and sprinkle with parsley. Serve warm.

Salsa dip

250g goat cheese

1 cup medium salsa

½ cup avocado, diced

1 green onion, sliced

2 pitas

2 tablespoons freshly ground flaxseeds

Preparation

Preheat the oven at 350ºF for 10 minutes.

Spread goat cheese on to a small oven pan and top with salsa and green onion. Bake for 10-15 minutes. Remove from heat. Add avocado and flaxseeds. Serve with pita wedges.

Brussels Sprouts-and-Brown Rice

1 lb (½ kg) Brussels sprouts
¼ cup water
1 tablespoon olive oil
2 tablespoons gluten free flour
1½ cups vegetable broth
salt and pepper, to taste
Cooking spray
1 cup wild rice , cooked
2 tablespoons goat cheese
1 cup of pecans, chopped

Preparation

1. Preheat oven to 375°F (190°C).

2. In a saucepan, add the Brussels sprouts, covered with water. Bring to a boil. Drain.

3. In another pan, heat the oil and add flour, while stirring. Add vegetable broth, salt and pepper and bring to a boil, stirring constantly.

4. Coat an oven pan with cooking spray. Place the rice at the bottom and Brussels sprouts on top. Pour the flour sauce and. Bake at 375°F until lightly browned.

5. Remove pan from oven, add goat cheese and pecans.

Kale and Tortilla Chips with Salsa

8 servings

1 bunch kale

200-225 grams (half bag) baked tortilla chips

2 tablespoons olive oil

1 tablespoon sesame seeds

salt and pepper, to taste

1 cup medium salsa

Preparation

1. Preheat oven to 300°F (148°C). Rinse kale, remove the ribs. Dry the leaves with paper towel. Tear leaves into small pieces.

2. Pour oil into a large bowl, add kale, and toss to coat evenly.

3. In a large oven pan, add the leaves. Bake, switching pan positions after 10 minutes. Sprinkle with sesame seeds, add tortilla chips and bake until kale leaves are crisp (but not browned). Serve with salsa.

Papaya Avocado Salsa Salad

4 servings (cups)

2 cups papaya, diced (keep & crush the seeds – two teaspoons)

2 ripe avocado, peeled, pitted & diced

2 tablespoons fresh cilantro, chopped

⅔ cup medium salsa

⅓ cup cucumbers, diced

Lemon juice (2 lemons)

Orange juice (½ orange)

Salt and pepper, to taste

Preparation

Mix the papaya, avocado, olive oil, salsa, and lemon, orange juice in a bowl. Add salt and pepper, to taste. Sprinkle with cilantro and crushed papaya seeds.

Brussels sprouts – Kale Salad

4 servings

½ bunch kale, keep the leaves only; chopped

1 pound Brussels Sprouts , sliced

1 red bell pepper diced

1 tablespoon olive oil

lime juice (use 1 lime)

¼ pumpkin seeds

¼ cup dried cranberries

¼ cup pecans, finely chopped

¼ cup sesame seeds

Preparation

Mix the Brussels sprouts, kale, red pepper (either fresh or lightly steamed) and cranberries. Toss to combine, add the olive oil and the lime juice, and toss again.

In a pan, toast the seeds over medium heat- first add the pumpkin seeds, then pecans; reduce temperature and add sesame seeds.

Add the seeds mixture to the salad and serve.

Quinoa Tabbouleh

6 servings

¾ cup quinoa

one bunch fresh parsley leaves, chopped

½ bunch fresh mint leaves, chopped

3 tomatoes, finely diced

one cup cucumbers, diced

2 scallions, finely chopped

2 tablespoons avocado oil

⅓ cup lime juice

Preparation

1. Prepare quinoa. Place quinoa (¾ cup) in a pan with water (1½ cups). Bring to a boil, cover, and simmer over low heat. Simmer until all liquid is absorbed. Remove from heat and let stand for 5 minutes.

2. Place quinoa, parsley, mint, tomato, cucumbers and scallions in a bowl. Toss to combine. Drizzle avocado oil and lime juice, add salt and pepper to taste and serve.

Alternative: in a pan coated with cooking spray add scallions, tomatoes and cucumbers and cook them for 5 minutes over low heat. Combine with parsley and mint. Add avocado oil and lime juice. Toss to combine. Mix with quinoa and serve.

Home Made Cheese

1 Gallon (3.78L) 3% Milk

¼ cup white vinegar

¼ cup lemon juice

Salt to taste

¼ cup sun dried tomatoes – optional

1 tablespoon oregano – optional

2 tablespoons olive oil

Preparation

Place milk into a large pot over medium heat, until tiny bubbles appear, right before it boils. Stir in vinegar or lemon and remove from heat. It will start to curdle. Pour cheese into cloth lined bowl. Bring together all four corners of cloth and twist around a spoon. Hang dripping cheese for a 1-2 hours. Add salt, olive oil (optional: dried tomatoes, oregano) and toss to combine. Refrigerate 20 min-1 hour before serving.

Polenta and Goat Cheese

4 servings

4 cups water
salt, to taste
1 teaspoon olive oil
1 cup cornmeal
4 tablespoons goat cheese

Preparation

In a saucepan, add water, olive oil and salt. Bring to a boil.

Stir in the cornmeal slowly and constantly, using a wooden spoon. Reduce temperature to low-medium and continue to stir until the polenta is thick. Place polenta in small bowls while hot. Add goat cheese.

Oven Potatoes and Salmon Fillet

4 servings

1 pound salmon fillet, cut into 4 portions
marinade: lime zest (one lime), 1 tablespoon olive oil,
1 teaspoon parsley flakes, dried and salt
salt and pepper, to taste
lime wedges
2 tablespoons leeks, chopped
2 large potatoes, peeled and cut into wedges
1 tablespoon olive oil

Preparation

1. Preheat oven to 425°F (218°C). Coat an oven pan with cooking spray.

2. In a small bowl prepared the marinade: lime zest (1 lime), 1 tablespoon olive oil, 1 teaspoon dried parsley, dash of salt and pepper. Add the salmon. Marinade for 10 minutes.

3. Place salmon in the oven pan.

4. Season with salt and pepper, then sprinkle with leeks. Cover with foil and bake until starting to flake.

5. In a second oven pan, coated with cooking spray place potatoes wedges. Add one tablespoon olive oil and sprinkle one teaspoon thyme. Potatoes may cook faster if the salmon fillets are thick.

6. When ready, place the salmon and potatoes to dinner plates. Serve with lemon wedges.

Roasted Turkey with Cranberry

4 servings

2 lb (1 kg) turkey breast
1 tablespoon olive oil
½ cup millet
salt and pepper , to taste
½ cup fresh cranberries
½ cup walnuts, chopped
1 tablespoon parsley flakes, dried

Preparation

Cooking millet: In a saucepan, bring 2 cups of water to a boil. Add millet and ½ tablespoon olive oil. Stir frequently. Cover and simmer over medium heat until millet becomes fluffy and the water is absorbed.

Cooking turkey

Heat oven to 450° F (232°C)

Rinse the turkey inside and dry with paper towel. Place in an oven pan.

Rub the oil over the skin. Add salt, pepper, parsley flakes and cranberries. Roast for 20 minutes. You may add ½ cup water and continue to roast until the meat is fully cooked.

Remove pan from the oven. Sprinkle with walnuts and serve with millet.

Chicken Thighs With Spinach and Penne

4 servings

10 oz. pasta (penne – choose gluten free)
1 bunch fresh spinach
salt and pepper, to taste
1½ pound chicken thighs
3 tablespoons olive oil
1 cup tomatoes, diced
4 tablespoons goat cheese

Preparation

Prepare penne according to package directions. Drain; return to pan. Stir in spinach; cover and keep warm over low heat.

Coat an oven pan with cooking spray. Add the chicken thighs. Add 1 tablespoon olive oil, salt and pepper and cook over medium-high heat until lightly browned.

Remove from oven and pour over pasta with spinach.

Pour over warm pasta mixture and goat cheese; toss to combine.

Transfer to a serving dish, and sprinkle with fresh tomatoes.

Curry Chicken with Ginger

4 servings

3 cups chicken breast, cut into strips

1 cup potatoes, diced

1 cup red bell peppers, sliced

3 tablespoons olive oil

½ teaspoon curry powder

salt and pepper, to taste

1 tablespoon fresh ginger, grated

Preparation

In a small bowl prepared the marinade: 2 tablespoons olive oil, curry powder, fresh ginger, dash of salt and pepper. Add the chicken breasts. Marinade for 10 minutes.

Coat an oven pan with cooking spray. Add the chicken breast. Add potatoes (aside of meat), pour 1 tablespoon olive oil, salt and pepper and cook over medium-high heat until chicken is lightly browned. Remove pan from the oven and serve.

Spaghetti Squash

4 servings

1 pound spaghetti squash
garlic clove, chopped
one small onion, chopped
3 medium Portobello mushrooms, sliced
1 green bell pepper, sliced
2 tomatoes, sliced
1 tablespoon Italian seasoning mix (rosemary, thyme and oregano)
cooking oil
one tablespoon olive oil
salt and pepper, to taste
4 tablespoons shredded low fat feta cheese

Preparation

Preheat oven to 375ºF (180ºC). Slice the squash in half lengthwise and remove the seeds. Place the squash into an oven pan coated with cooking oil. Bake it face-down until easily pierced by a fork (around 30 minutes). Remove it from the oven.

In a saucepan, add one tablespoon of oil and bring to a heat. Saute the tomatoes, onions, garlic, green pepper and mushrooms, Italian seasoning mix (oregano, thyme and rosemary). Add salt and pepper to taste.

Scoop out spaghetti squash pulp, using a fork, and scrap out flesh. It should come out in spaghetti like ribbons.

Transfer to a serving dish. Add sautéed vegetables and sprinkle with feta cheese.

Curried Cauliflower & Chickpea

4-6 servings

1 tablespoon olive oil
½ lb (225 g) turkey breasts, cut into ½-inch pieces
1 onion, chopped
2 cloves garlic, chopped
4 teaspoons gingerroot, grated
2 teaspoons curry powder
3 cups cauliflower florets
1 cup tomatoes, diced
1 cup chickpeas, canned and drained
¼ cup water
⅓ cup chopped cilantro

Preparation

Heat the olive oil in large pan on medium-high heat. Add turkey, onions and garlic and cook until meat is tender. Add ginger, curry powder, cauliflower, tomatoes and chickpea. Add water and bring to a boil and cook until the turkey is fully cooked and the veggies are soften. Remove from heat, sprinkle cilantro and serve.

Greek Kabobs

16 skewers

Dressing
½ cup olive oil
1 teaspoon oregano
1 teaspoon thyme
2 tablespoon lime juice
salt and pepper, to taste
1 tablespoon olive oil
1½ lb (675 g) chicken breasts, cut into small cubes
1 red onion, cut into small wedges
1 lemon, sliced (round slices)
2 avocado, pitted, peeled and diced
3 large tomatoes, diced

Preparation
In a bowl, mix the oil with oregano, thyme and a dash of salt. Pour the dressing over chicken. Marinate for 15-20 minutes.

Heat the barbeque and thread chicken alternating with onions onto sixteen skewers. Place the lemon slices on the barbecue for one minute, and serve them next to kabobs.

In a bowl mix avocado and tomatoes. Add 1 tablespoon lime juice, 1 tablespoon olive oil, salt and pepper. Serve with kabobs.

Onion, Olive and Red Pepper Tart

Serves 6

2 large onions, sliced

4 sheets of gluten free phyllo

½ cup goat cheese

12 cup pitted kalamata olives, cut in half

1 red bell pepper, sliced

1 tablespoon chopped fresh thyme

salt and pepper, to taste

1 tablespoon olive oil

Preparation

Preheat oven to 400°F (204°C).

In a sauce pan, add the olive oil and bring to a heat. Add onions and sauté. Remove from heat.

Add the first phyllo sheet to a cooking pan coated with cooking oil. Spray each phyllo sheets with cooking spray, and add one sheet on top to another. Top the phyllo with goat cheese, olives, red peppers and cooked onions. Bake until the phyllos are cooked (10-15 minutes). Sprinkle with thyme and serve.

Thai Kabobs

16 skewers

Dressing:
½ cup vegetable broth
¼ cup honey
3 tablespoons soy sauce
1 garlic clove, chopped
2 red bell peppers, cut in square pieces
½ lb (675 g) chicken breasts, cut into small cubes.
One bag of rice crackers

Preparation

In a bowl, mix the broth with honey, soy sauce and garlic. Pour the dressing over chicken. Marinate for 15-20 minutes.

Heat the barbeque and thread chicken alternating with bell peppers onto sixteen skewers. Serve with rice crackers.

Vegetarian Tacos

4 portions (8 small tacos)

1 tablespoon olive oil
1 cup of tempeh, diced
2 cups of mixed frozen vegetables (corn, pea and carrots)
1 garlic clove, minced
8 small corn tortilla
¾ cup medium salsa
salt and pepper, to taste
¾ cup feta cheese, crumbled
optional: green mixed salad

Preparation

Heat one tablespoon olive oil in a pan, over medium heat. Add frozen vegetables and garlic clove and brings to a heat. Add tempeh, salt and pepper and cook until vegetables are soft and tempeh becomes golden brown. Remove from heat.

Fill tortillas with tempeh mixture, add feta cheese and salsa (adding green mix salad optional) and serve.

Vegetarian Burger

6 burgers

3 portobello mushrooms, sliced
1 onion, sliced
3 tablespoons olive oil
one garlic clove
salt and pepper, to taste
1 cup black beans, canned, drained
½ cup of frozen corn
½ cup carrots, shredded
½ cup tomato sauce
2 eggs
6 small aluminum pie pans

Preparation

Heat a pan coated with cooking oil, over medium heat. Add onion and garlic and sauté. Add mushrooms and cook until tender. Transfer to a bowl.

Place the frozen corn in the same pan, and cook for few minutes, until warm.

In a large pan mix the mushroom mixture with eggs, corn, black beans, carrots, tomato sauce, salt and pepper. Toss to combine and cook for 15 minutes. Remove from heat and place this mixture into small aluminum pie pans. Cool and refrigerate or place the burgers in the oven to cook them.

Lemon Dijon Chicken

4 servings

4 skinless, boneless chicken breast – cut into small strips
½ lime juice
1 lemon, juice
3 tablespoons Dijon mustard
salt and pepper to taste
one tablespoon fresh parsley leaves
one avocado, peeled, pitted and sliced
one orange, peeled and sliced
cooking oil
1 tablespoon olive oil
one tablespoon fresh ground flaxseeds

Preparation

Heat a pan coated with cooking oil, over medium heat. Place chicken, lime and lemon juice, mustard, salt, pepper, and parsley and cook until done (10-15 minutes).

In a bowl, mix together avocado and orange. Add one teaspoon olive oil. Sprinkle with flax seeds. Serve with Dijon chicken.

Chicken Pesto with Mashed Potatoes

4 boneless skinless chicken breasts

½ cup basil pesto

1 large tomato

4 potatoes, peeled and diced

one tablespoon olive oil

½ cup yogurt

½ tablespoon fresh parsley leaves

salt and pepper, to taste

cooking spray

Preparation

Preheat oven to 400°F (204°C).

In a saucepan place the potatoes in water and cook until tender. Drain. Mash potatoes with a fork. Add yogurt, salt and pepper, and top with fresh parsley leaves.

Place pesto and chicken in bowl and toss until chicken is fully covered.

Place the chicken in an oven pan coated with cooking spray. Add tomato slices on top. Bake until chicken is fully cooked (20-30 minutes). Remove from oven and serve with mashed potatoes.

Halibut in Tomato Sauce with Asparagus

2 tablespoons olive oil

4 halibut fillets

one garlic clove

one small onion, sliced

½ cup kalamata olives, pitted and sliced

1 cup tomatoes, diced

one teaspoon basil

one teaspoon oregano

salt and pepper, to taste

1 lb fresh asparagus spears, trimmed

1 tablespoon ground flax seeds

1 teaspoon lemon juice

lime wedges

Preparation

Heat 1 tablespoon olive oil in a pan over medium heat. Add garlic and onion and sauté. Add one cup of water, tomatoes, basil and oregano and bring to a boil. Reduce heat and add the fish. Cook until fish flakes. Remove from heat and cover the pan.

In a second pan heat ½ tablespoon olive oil over medium heat. Add asparagus and cook until is tender. Remove from heat, add the remaining ½ tablespoon of olive oil, lemon juice, salt and pepper. Serve with halibut and lime wedges.

Asparagus Risotto with Tuna Fish

½ onion, chopped

1½ tablespoon olive oil

1 cup brown rice, uncooked

1 lb (½ kg) fresh asparagus spears, cut into small pieces

1 cup vegetable broth

2 tablespoons goat cheese

lemon zest from 1 lemon

orange zest from ¼ orange

2 cans tuna fish

salt and pepper, to taste

one tablespoon fresh parsley leaves

Preparation

Heat 1 tablespoon olive oil in a pan over medium heat. Add onion and sauté. Add rice, asparagus and broth, while stirring. Bring to a boil. Reduce heat and cook until rice is soft. Add goat cheese, half of lemon and orange zest, salt and pepper.

In a bowl, mix tuna fish with ½ tablespoon olive oil, the remaining lemon and oranges zest and fresh parsley. Serve with rice.

Crab Cakes with Salad

Serves 4

1 pound crabmeat (remove shells)

⅓ cup rice crackers

3 green onions, chopped

½ cup red bell pepper, chopped

½ tomatoes, diced

1 egg

2 tablespoons gluten free flour

one tablespoon lemon juice

one garlic clove

salt and pepper, to taste

Flour, for dusting

2 tablespoons olive

3 cups green salad

In a large bowl, mix the crabmeat with crushed rice crackers, bell pepper, tomatoes, egg, garlic, lemon juice, salt and pepper. Divide the mixture into 6 patties. Cover the patties with flour.

Heat olive oil in a pan over medium heat. Place the crab cakes and cook until golden brown on each side. Serve with green salad.

Scallops with Cabbage Salad

4 servings

1 lb (½ kg) scallops
2 tablespoons olive oil
1 tablespoon balsamic vinegar
salt and pepper, to taste
¼ medium red cabbage, chopped

Preparation

Remove the small side muscle from the scallops.

Heat 1 tablespoon olive oil in a pan over medium heat. Add the scallops, salt and pepper and cook few minutes on each side, until a golden crust forms.

In a bowl place the cabbage, and add one tablespoon of balsamic vinegar, one tablespoon of olive oil, salt and pepper. Serve with scallops.

Shrimp Dinner

2 cups vegetable broth

4 tablespoons gluten free flour

½ cup goat cheese

1 red bell pepper, finely sliced

1 zucchini, finely diced

one pound (½ kg) shrimp

¾ cup bread crumbs (gluten free), crushed

one garlic clove, chopped

cooking spray

Preparation

Preheat oven to 350ºF (176ºC).

In a saucepan, combine the vegetable broth with flour and bring to a boil. Add the goat cheese, red pepper, zucchini and garlic.

In an oven pot coated with cooking spray add the shrimps. Pour the flour mixture, and then top with bread crumbs. Bake in the oven for 40 minutes, or until the shrimps are fully cooked. Cool before serving.

Turkey Meatballs

4 servings

2 tablespoons olive oil
one onion, finely chopped
2 garlic cloves, finely chopped
1 tablespoon fresh parsley, chopped
½ cup tomato sauce
⅓ cup bread (gluten free) crumbs
one pound (½ kg) ground turkey
1 egg
salt and pepper, to taste
Cooking spray
2 cups mixed frozen vegetables (pea, carrots, corn)

Preparation

Preheat oven at 400ºF (204ºC).

Heat 1 tablespoon olive oil in a pan over medium heat. Add onion and garlic, and sauté.

Soak bread crumbs in tomato sauce. Add ground turkey, cooked onion and garlic onions, parsley and egg, salt and pepper. Mix until smooth.

Shape into small balls and place them in an oven pan coated with cooking spray. Bake until the meat if fully cooked (around 30 minutes).

In another pan, heat 1 tablespoon olive oil in a pan over medium heat. Add frozen vegetables and cook until warm. Add salt and pepper and serve with meatballs.

Snacks

Granola Bars

10 bars

3½ cups gluten free cereals
¾ cup applesauce
¼ cup honey
¼ cup light molasses
½ cup pecans, chopped
¼ cup pumpkin seeds
¼ cup raisins
1 teaspoon cinnamon

Preparation

Heat oven to 325°F (162ºC). Line 8-inch square pan with parchment paper, extending paper over sides of pan, and line cookie sheet with parchment paper.

Place the cereals in a food processor and pulse for one minute to break down in small pieces. Transfer them into a large bowl. Add applesauce, honey, molasses, cinnamon, pecans, pumpkin seeds and raisins. Toss to combine.

Pour this mixture into an oven pan coated with cooking spray. Press this mixture so it covers completely the bottom of the pan. Bake for 20-30 minutes (depending whether you prefer soft or crunchy bars). Cool for few minutes before cutting into bars. Refrigerate before serving.

Fruity Yogurt

4 servings

2 cups plain yogurt
1 teaspoon cinnamon
1 tablespoon honey
¼ cup blueberries
¼ cup dried apricots
1 tablespoon fresh grounded flax seeds

Preparation

In a bowl mix the yogurt with blueberries, apricots and honey.

Top with cinnamon and flax seeds and serve.

Veggie Yogurt

4 servings

2 cups plain yogurt
1 tablespoon parsley leaves, chopped
¼ cup of baby carrots, sliced (round slices)
¼ cup of cucumbers, diced (small dices)
¼ cup of red bell pepper, sliced
2 tablespoons sesame seeds, roasted
salt, to taste

Preparation

Roast the sesame seeds in a dry, oil free pan over low heat, for 2-3 minutes, stirring often.

In a bowl, mix the yogurt with carrots, parsley, cucumbers and red peppers.

Top with sesame seeds, add salt to taste.

Nutty Yogurt

4 servings

2 cups plain yogurt
2 tablespoons pumpkin seeds
2 tablespoons walnuts, chopped
2 tablespoons pine nuts
1 tablespoon fresh grounded flax seeds
salt, to taste

Preparation

Roast the pumpkin seeds, walnuts and pine nuts in a dry, oil free pan, over low heat for 5-7 minutes, stirring often.

In a bowl, mix the yogurt with nuts and seeds. Add salt to taste. Top with flax seeds.

Apple Banana Toast

4 servings

4 slices gluten free bread
1 apples, cored and sliced
½ banana sliced
1 tablespoon coconut oil
1 tablespoon ground cinnamon
½ tablespoon brown sugar.

Preparation

Preheat the oven 325ºF (162ºC).

Place bread slices into an oven pan. Spread coconut oil on one side of each slice of bread. Add apple and banana slices. Top with cinnamon and sugar. Bake for 10 minutes. Serve warm.

Protein Rich Snack 1

4 servings

8 white eggs

2 eggs

1 Portobello mushroom, finely sliced

Salt and pepper to taste

2 dill pickled cucumber, diced

1 tablespoon fresh dill

cooking spray

Preparation

Whisk the eggs, white eggs in a bowl.

Heat a pan over medium heat. Add the egg mixture and Portobello mushroom and stir with a spatula to scramble, until cooked.

Transfer the egg mixture to a bowl. Add pickled cucumbers and salt and pepper, to taste. Sprinkle with fresh dill.

Protein Rich Snack 2

4 servings

1 cup of mixed canned beans, drained

½ cup of black olives, pitted and sliced

½ cup white mushrooms, canned

1 tablespoon olive oil

1 tablespoon lime juice

salt and pepper, to taste

½ tablespoon Italian mix dried herbs (oregano, rosemary, thyme)

1 tablespoon sesame seeds

Preparation

In a bowl, mix the beans, olives, mushrooms, sesame seeds and olive oil. Add salt, pepper and Italian mix herbs and toss to combine.

Heat a pan over medium heat. Add this mixture and cook for 5 minutes. Remove from heat. Add lemon juice. Serve.

Protein Rich Snack 3

4 servings

½ lb (¼ kg) smoked turkey thigh, cut into small strips
½ cup green olives
2 boiled eggs, sliced
½ cup sauerkraut
salt and pepper, to taste

Preparation

In a bowl, mix the turkey, olives, eggs and sauerkraut. Add salt and pepper and toss to combine and serve.

Protein Rich Snack 4

4 servings

2 cans tuna fish, drained
1 green bell pepper, finely diced
¼ cup kalamata olives, pitted and sliced
½ cup of avocado, peeled, pitted and diced
½ cup of yogurt
salt and pepper, to taste
1 tablespoon flax seeds, freshly grounded
1 tablespoon lime juice

Preparation

In a bowl, mix tuna fish with pepper, olives and yogurt. Add salt and pepper and toss to combine. Top with avocado. Sprinkle with flax seeds and drizzle lime juice.

Desserts

Cheese Triangles

8 triangles

4 sheets gluten free phyllo
1 cup cottage cheese
¼ cup brown sugar
cooking spray
one tablespoon ground cinnamon

Preparation

Preheat oven to 400°F (204ºC). Spray 1 each phyllo sheets with cooking spray, and add one sheet on top to another. Cut crosswise the phyllos into eight equal strips.

In a bowl, mix cottage cheese with brown sugar. Spoon one teaspoon of cheese onto the bottom corner of each strip. Fold the end of the dough over cottage cheese to form a triangle. Continue to fold the same way the entire length of the dough. Repeat with the remaining phyllo strips. Place each strip in an oven pan coated with cooking spray. Bake for 7-10 minutes. Sprinkle with cinnamon and serve.

Pecan Tarts

6 tarts

¼ cup gluten free flour

½ coconut oil, melted

¼ cup cream cheese

¼ cup raisins

¼ cup pecans, chopped

¼ cup honey

½ teaspoon natural vanilla

1 egg

Preparation

Place the flour, coconut oil and cream cheese in food processor and mix until well blended . Shape this mixture into small balls with hands; wrap the balls with plastic wrap and place them in the fridge for one hour.

Heat the oven to 375ºF (190ºC). Roll out pastry on lightly floured surface. Divide into 6 small rounds cutter. Place them in muffin cups coated with cooking spray. Top them with raisins and pecans. Beat lightly the egg, mix with vanilla and honey and spoon over the tarts. Bake until lightly browned (15-18 min).

Peach-Raspberry Cake

6 servings (pieces)

Cake:

¾ cups gluten free flour

1 teaspoons gluten free baking powder

dash of baking soda & dash of salt

⅓ cup brown sugar

1 tablespoon coconut oil

1 egg

1 tablespoon raspberry jam

½ cup almond milk

1 cup peaches sliced

1teaspoon lemon zest finely shredded

Cooking spray

Topping:

1 tablespoon brown sugar

2 tablespoons walnuts, finely chopped

1 tablespoons coconut oil

½ teaspoon ground cinnamon

Preparation

Preheat oven to 350ºF (176ºC).

To prepare cake: In another bowl, mix brown sugar with 2 tablespoons coconut oil, egg and raspberry juice, using a mixer-until blended well. Add flour, backing powder, backing soda, salt, almond milk and peaches and mix well with a wooden spoon. Add this mixture to a baking pan coated with cooking spray.

To prepare topping: Mix sugar, walnuts, cinnamon and coconut oil with a wooden spoon, until moist. Sprinkle over batter. Bake at 350°F until a wooden pick inserted in center comes out clean.

Home Made Vanilla Ice Cream

Serves 4

1 cup (raw) pecans, chopped
2 cups low fat yogurt
¼ cup agave nectar
1 tablespoon natural vanilla extract
1 cup fresh berries

Preparation

Mix all ingredients in a bowl and blend on high speed.

Pour the content in a freezer bowl and refrigerate 2-3 hours.

Serve with fresh berries.

Plum and Rhubarb Crisp

6 servings

2½ cups sliced plums

2 cups sliced rhubarb

⅓ cup brown sugar

1½ tablespoons gluten free flour

Cooking spray

½ cup old-fashioned rolled oats

¼ cup brown sugar

½ cup gluten free flour

dash of salt

1 tablespoon coconut oil

2 cups home made vanilla ice cream

Preparation

1. Mix fruits with ⅓ cup sugar and 1½ tablespoon flour in a bowl.

2. Preheat oven to 400°F.

3. Add this mixture to a baking pan coated with cooking spray. Bake at 400ºF for until bubbly (30-35 min)

4. Mix oats with flour and sugar in a bowl. Add coconut oil. Sprinkle oat mixture over fruit. Bake until topping is lightly browned and fruit is bubbly (10-15 min). Serve warm with ice cream.

Lemon Pound Cake with Peaches

8 servings

1 cup gluten free flour
¼ cup cornmeal
½ teaspoon gluten free baking soda
dash of salt
¾ cups brown sugar
5 tablespoon coconut oil
2 eggs yolks and 2 egg whites
1 teaspoons finely shredded lemon zest
½ teaspoon natural vanilla extract
⅓ cup almond milk
1½ tablespoons fresh lemon juice
1 cup of fresh peaches, sliced
Cooking spray

Preparation

Preheat oven to 350°F.

Mix flour with baking soda and cornmeal in a bowl

In another bowl, mix brown sugar with coconut oil with a wooden spoon until fluffy.

Add egg yolks, lemon zest, lemon juice and vanilla and blend them well. Pour in the flour mixture

Place egg whites in a bowl and beat at high speed until stiff peaks form.

Add slowly egg whites into batter, then add peaches. Add this mixture to a baking pan coated with cooking spray. Bake at 350ºF until wooden pick inserted in center comes out clean.

Orange Curd with Mango

Serves 4

½ cup sugar

½ cup fresh orange juice

pinch of salt

3 egg yolks

½ tablespoons coconut oil

teaspoons finely shredded orange zest

1½ cups fresh mango, peeled and diced

¼ cup walnuts, chopped

Preparation

1. Mix sugar, orange juice, egg yolks and salt in a saucepan over medium heat, stir constantly until thick. Add coconut oil and orange zest. The orange curd will be ready when it coats a spoon. Remove from heat.

2. Place curd in a bowl, cover and chill completely.

3. Spoon 2 tablespoons curd into cups. Top each serving with mango and chopped walnuts.

Coffee Cake

Serves 6–8

⅓ cup unsweetened applesauce

1 cup brown sugar

2 eggs

1 cup gluten free flour

dash of salt

2 teaspoon gluten free baking powder

1 cup yogurt

1 tablespoon vanilla

2 tablespoon cinnamon

½ cup brown sugar

2 tablespoons coconut oil.

Cooking spray

Preparation

Add applesauce, 1 cup brown sugar to a bowl and thoroughly combine with an electric mixer medium-high speed. Add eggs, vanilla, flour, baking soda and yogurt. Stir.

Preheat oven to 350°F. Combine remaining ½ cup sugar with one tablespoon coconut oil and cinnamon.

Pour batter into the pan coated with cooking spray. Add the sugar-coconut oil mixture on top. Bake at 350°F until wooden pick inserted in center comes out clean (50 minutes or so).

Applesauce Lemon Biscotti

24 biscotti

1½ tablespoons coconut oil

5 tablespoons applesauce, unsweetened

½ cup sugar, 2 eggs

teaspoon natural vanilla

½ tablespoon orange zest finely shredded

1½ tablespoons lemon zest finely shredded

2 cups gluten free flour, dash of salt

teaspoon gluten free baking powder

Cooking spray

Preparation

Add applesauce, coconut oil, and sugar to a bowl and thoroughly combine with an electric mixer medium-high speed. Add the eggs, vanilla, lemon zest and continue to mix.

Add flour, salt, and baking powder, using a wooden spoon to blend all the ingredients, until a dough forms. Divide the dough into two log shape pieces.

Place doughs into the oven pan coated with cooking spray. Bake at 350°F for 30 minutes. Remove the biscotti logs from the oven and let them cool before cutting them into slices. Place biscotti slices again in the oven for 5 more minutes.

Peach and Blueberry Tart

10 servings

1 cup ricotta cheese
½ cup + 2 tablespoons brown sugar
2 teaspoons salt
2 teaspoons orange zest finely shredded
1 egg
1 cup ground pecans + 1 tablespoon sliced pecans
1½ teaspoons ground cinnamon
6 sheets phyllo dough
2 tablespoons coconut oil
8 peaces, sliced
1 cup fresh blueberries
Cooking spray

Preparation

1. Preheat oven to 400°F (204°C) with rack in the center.
2. Mix ricotta, ½ cup sugar, salt, egg, and ground walnuts in a bowl.
3. In another bowl, mix cinnamon, orange zest with 2 tablespoons sugar.
4. Place the first phyllo dough into the oven pan coated with cooking spray. Brush it phyllo dough with coconut oil, using a brush pastry. Sprinkle with cinnamon, orange zest and sugar. Layer, brush and sprinkle the remaining phyllo sheets, one on top of the other.
5. Spread evenly ricotta on top of the phyllo sheets. Add peaches, blueberries and sliced walnuts. Bake at 400°C until the crust is golden brown.

Power Waffle

One serving (waffle)

1 frozen gluten free waffle.
1 teaspoon coconut oil
½ cup blueberries
½ cup banana slices
1 teaspoon walnuts sliced
1 teaspoon agave nectar

Preparation

Toast the waffle. Spread it with coconut butter. Top with blueberries and banana; sprinkle walnuts and drizzle with agave nectar.

Crunchy Parfait with Raspberries and Apricots

8 servings

Cooking spray
½ cup packed light brown sugar
4 tablespoons coconut oil
1 cup gluten free rolled oats
¾ cup mixed almonds, pecans, walnuts, sliced
4 cups low fat yogurt
1 cup raspberries
2 cups apricots, diced
1 tablespoon ground cinnamon.

Preparation

Preheat oven to 350°F (176°C).

In a saucepan, heat brown sugar and cooking oil. Stir. Remove from heat and add the oats, almonds and walnuts. Place this mixture into an oven pan coated with cooking spray. Bake until golden and crunchy. Crumble into small pieces.

In small bowls add the crunch, yogurt and fruits in layers. Sprinkle with cinnamon.

Shortbread Cookies

18 cookies

1½ cups gluten free flour
⅔ cup sugar
¼ cup tapioca
1 tablespoon orange zest, shredded
dash of salt
6 tablespoons coconut oil
⅔ cup mixed nuts: almonds, walnuts, pecans
Cooking spray

Preparation

Preheat oven to 350°F (176°C).

Mix flour, tapioca, sugar, lemon zest and salt in a food processor. Place this mixture in a bowl and add coconut oil. Stir in the nuts. Place 4 tablespoon of mixture into each muffin cup coated with cooking spray (if you use regular muffin cups, you will get 18 cookies). Bake until wooden pick inserted in center comes out clean.

Cranberry-Citrus Muffins

6 muffins

¾ cup chopped cranberries

1 cup + 1 tablespoons gluten free flour

¼ cup brown sugar

1 teaspoon gluten free baking powder

dash of teaspoon salt

4 tablespoons coconut oil

½ teaspoon orange zest finely shredded

¼ teaspoon ground cinnamon

2 eggs

1 cup low-fat yogurt

Cooking spray

1½ teaspoons honey

Preparation

1. Preheat oven to 375°F (190°C).

2. Mix flour, sugar, baking powder, and salt in a bowl.

3. In another bowl mix 2 cup flour coconut oil, orange zest, cinnamon, eggs, yogurt with a wooden spoon. Add cranberries.

4. Spoon the batter into 12 muffin cups (regular size) coated with cooking spray. Add honey on top. Bake at 375°F until wooden pick inserted in center comes out clean.

Gluten Free Carrot Cake

18 muffin cups

1 cups brown sugar

2 eggs

¾ cup coconut oil, melted + 4 tablespoons

1 cups gluten-free flour

1 teaspoon baking soda

1 teaspoons gluten-free baking powder

1½ teaspoons cinnamon

dash of salt

1 teaspoon natural vanilla extract

½ cup pecans, chopped

1½ cups carrots, grated

Preparation

Mix sugar and eggs in a large mixing bowl with an electric beater or stand mixer. Add oil and vanilla and beat just until smooth.

In a bowl mix the flour mix, baking soda, baking powder and salt, using a whisk. Add eggs, brown sugar and yogurt and whisk to combine. Add carrots and nuts.

Pour the mixture into the muffin cups. Bake until a toothpick inserted in the cake comes out clean (around 30 minutes).

Baked Apples

6 servings

6 apples – peeled, seeds removed
1 tablespoon brown sugar
1 tablespoon ground cinnamon
¼ cup raisins
¼ cup pecans, chopped
cooking oil

Preparation

Preheat oven to 350°F (176°C).

Place the apples in an oven pan coated with cooking oil.

In a bowl mix the sugar, cinnamon, raisins and pecans.

Fill the apples with this mixture. Cook until apples are soft and bubbly (45-60 minutes). Serve.